Praise for Steve Agren

CW00662154

"As a cardiothoracic surgeon ca
regular basis, I have had an opp
ly with Steve Agren. Steve has
in all aspects of atrial fibrillatio......
risks factors as well as all of the latest treatment options.
Steve's warm, outgoing nature and personal experience
with afib give him great insight into helping others manage
their own afib. He is truly an expert in his field."

**Rafael Squitieri, MD, Founder, TURNCARE Pressure Ulcer Management Solutions,
Chief of Cardiothoracic Surgery, St. Vincent's Medical Center, Bridgeport, CT**

"Steve is intelligent, diligent, thoughtful, very organized,
hardworking, and he always has the patient in mind with
everything he does. He also has the insight and first-hand
knowledge to understand Afib and the way it can affect people and what all the potential options are for treatment."

**Kourosh T. Asgarian, DO, FACS,
Cardiothoracic Surgeon, Morristown Memorial Hospital, Morristown, NJ**

"Thanks to the knowledge and inspiration from AFstrokeRisk, I successfully quit smoking, reduced my alcohol
and caffeine consumption, improved my nutrition, and am
feeling better than ever! My family and I thank you!"

Danny Perry, Abington, PA

"Steve was always a tremendous asset both in the clinical
setting and in the operating room when treating atrial
fibrillation patients. His insight and knowledge base af-
forded me the ability to rely upon him as a colleague."

**Joseph Tiano, MD, FACC, Medical Director -
Electrophysiology Laboratory, St. Vincent's Medical Center, Bridgeport, CT**

AFstrokeRisk.com

"Steve has an incredible depth of knowledge about afib – both its causes and treatment. He has been a great asset to me as I have developed in my surgical treatment of afib. Any information that he provides is guaranteed to be up to date, cutting edge, and completely reliable."

Albert Dimeo, MD, Cardiothoracic Surgeon,
St. Francis Hospital, Roslyn, New York

"Steve, you were an amazing source of knowledge and comfort when I was first diagnosed with my heart PVC. I had no idea what the diagnosis meant for me, whether I should seek treatment or who I could even trust in the field. You took the time to reach out to me and explained what was happening to me in a very reassuring and informing way. Your explanation of what procedures were available, what those procedures looked like and most importantly your personal knowledge of the physicians, gave me the courage to seek the treatment I needed! I want to deeply thank you for walking me through a very scary time in my life."

Amiee R. Buckman, Esquire, Sarasota, FL

Mission
C·R·I·T·I·C·A·L

Mission
C·R·I·T·I·C·A·L

Manage your Atrial Fibrillation and Reduce your Risk of Stroke

Steve Agren

Copyright © 2017 by Steve Agren.

All rights reserved.

No part of this book may be used or reproduced in any manner whatsoever without written permission from the author. For information, address:

AFstrokeRisk, P.O. Box 15712, Sarasota, FL 34277

For more information about this book or the author, visit AFstrokeRisk.com

ISBN: 978-0-692-95598-7

Cover and Interior Design: DesignByIndigo.com

FIRST EDITION

Contents

DISCLAIMER

This Book Does Not Provide Medical Advice

The contents of this book including, but not limited to, the text, graphics, images and other material is provided for informational purposes only. The purpose of this book is to promote consumer understanding of various health topics including atrial fibrillation. It is not intended to be a substitute for professional medical advice, diagnosis or treatment. Always seek the advice of your physician or other qualified health care provider regarding a medical condition or treatment. Also seek the advice of your physician before undertaking a new health care regimen. Do not disregard professional medical advice or delay seeking such advice because of something you have read in this book.

Before starting any new diet or exercise program, consult with your doctor and clear any exercise and/or diet changes with them. I am not a doctor or a registered dietitian. I do not claim to diagnose, treat, prevent or cure any condition or disease. I do not provide medical aid or nutritional advice for the purpose of health or disease management. The information held in this book is merely the opinion of a layman. I am not a doctor, nor do I claim to have any formal medical background. I am not liable, either expressly or in an implied manner, nor do I have responsibility for any physical or emotional problems that may occur directly or indirectly from reading this book.

The information in this book is intended only to help you cooperate with your doctor, or wellness professional, in your efforts toward desirable health. Only your doctor can determine what is right for you. In addition to regular checkups and medical supervision, before starting any program that will impact your health, you should consult with your personal physician.

All information is generalized, presented for informational purposes only, not medical advice, and presented "as is" without warranty or guarantee of any kind. Readers are cautioned not to rely on this information as medical advice and to consult a qualified medical, dietary, fitness or other appropriate professional for their specific needs.

This information in this book has not been evaluated by the FDA or any other government agency and this information is not intended to "diagnose, treat, cure or prevent any disease."

Be smart. It's your body and your health.

Acknowledgements

This book would not have been possible without help, guidance, and support from many people. I am blessed to know each of you, and thank God our paths crossed.

Thank you to my best friend and wife, Beth, who provided the vision for this project. I truly appreciate your enduring love and patience. You made this seem easy, and helped make this dream come true. I want to thank our three amazing boys, Matthew, Oliver and Isaac – who are precious gifts that we are so fortunate to have in our life. You guys are my heroes and will go on to achieve greatness. And, of course, thank you to my parents for bringing me into the world and for shaping the personality that I rely on every day to reach higher and higher goals.

Thank you to Deana Tierney, Dr. Kourosh Asgarian, Rich Spinogatti, Dr. Charles Russo, and Audria Wooster, who all played a huge role in helping to refine this book. Your effort and passion blew me away in the moment, and even more so now that I reflect upon the process.

Thank you to Dr. Rafe Squitieri, Dr. Al DiMeo, and Dr. Joe Tiano – the trio I had the extreme pleasure of working with for years, who then ended up treating my AF and are now dear friends. And, thank you to all the other physicians, peers and colleagues, not specifically named; I want to express my sincere gratitude to all of you for your positive impact on my career and my knowledge of atrial fibrillation.

Finally, special thanks to *you* for choosing to read this book.

Love to all.

Introduction

" A wise man should consider that health
is the greatest of human blessings,
and learn how by his own thought to derive
benefit from his illnesses."

- Hippocrates

You have taken a step that could save your life. You know that your heart is what keeps your body, and many of its systems, working efficiently. Atrial fibrillation is a sign your system is not working correctly. Without a healthy heart, your entire system can fail. Mission Critical is a phrase used to describe any system where multiple factors can influence its survival or success. It is critical to know that every aspect of your life influences the health of your heart. It is not just diet and exercise, but rather that every experience you encounter has an effect on your heart. Mission Critical, in this book, details all the factors and how to approach them in order to manage your atrial fibrillation and reduce your risk of stroke.

It is critical to understand that winning this battle depends on you taking control back over your life, implementing the strategies in this book, and having the will-power and desire to live a healthy lifestyle.

When your life and health feel upside down, it is critical to be on a mission to explore the many possibilities that can reverse your path.

First, I would like to share a little bit about my journey, before setting you off on your mission...

It was a cold morning in December. I woke at 5 AM after a horrible night's sleep. My heart was thumping and pounding and it felt like it was going to jump out of my chest. I wondered "Is this a heart attack?" I got nervous and began to sweat profusely. I rolled on to my left side and tried to calm down, but lying on my left side seemed to make things worse and I remembered my heart is on that side of my body. The pounding seemed to echo into my left ear. As I rolled to my right side, my stress was mounting and I thought "I can't die...I have a beautiful wife lying next to me, three amazing boys, a great job, and 40 years left of life!"

I placed my fingers to my neck and took my pulse. As soon as I felt the rapid beat, I knew what was happening. It was atrial fibrillation (generally referred to as AF or afib).

How did I know? Most of my career has been spent working in the cardiac medical device industry, and focusing on AF. As a result, I have learned more about this condition than the average person. My occupation is selling specialized products to physicians and advising them as to the use of those products in the operating room for treatment of patients with AF. I have been present during close to a thousand cardiac procedures, and I have worked with some of the top surgeons, cardiologists and electrophysiologists in the world. My day consists of waking up, putting on my scrubs, and heading to the operating room or lab to help doctors who repair hearts so that they pump well and beat normally.

However, that particular morning at 5 AM, with a heart that felt ready to jump out of my chest, the thousands of conversations I've had with uber-intelligent doctors seemed to escape me. My mind was fuzzy and I was getting more and more frightened with every pounding beat.

I know very well that when you are experiencing AF, it is hard to make sense of anything. It's hard not to think about the hammering in your chest. It's hard not to feel like your life is about to end. It's hard not to think about your loved ones, and the possibility of leaving them. At that moment, it's hard not to shake with fear, worrying that you may have a stroke, and hard not to believe that at any second your heart could stop.

I feel blessed for all I have learned about AF over the years. I feel compelled to help you understand your AF and to help you understand how to reduce your risk of stroke, by sharing everything I know. I understand. I understand not only from a clinical point of view, but I understand because I, too, am battling AF.

The day I first experienced AF, I tried to push through and pretend all was normal. But by 10AM, I surrendered. My heart had been racing longer than during any marathon I had ever run. Having once been an elite athlete, I recognized that my body was extremely fatigued. By this point, my chest hurt, I was light-headed, totally exhausted, had a headache, heartburn and nausea, and I knew it was time to seek help.

In desperation, I called Dr. Kourosh Asgarian, who is a cardiac surgeon with whom I had worked for years. He urged me to go to the ER at a hospital near where I lived. When I arrived at the hospital, I was quickly assigned a room and another cardiac surgeon with whom I had worked closely, Dr. Rafael Squitieri, examined me within minutes. My heart rate was elevated to an abnormally high 185 beats per minute, which meant my heart had beat more than 50,000 times since 5 AM. Another colleague, Dr. Joe Tiano, an electrophysiologist, prescribed a medicine to be administered intravenously. Within 15 minutes I felt my heart return to its normal rhythm. I was lucky. If the medicine hadn't helped, they would have given me an electric shock called cardioversion.

My life was saved that day, and I was changed forever.

I decided that this terrifying experience should become a positive force in my life. It was time to take all the knowledge and information I had gained over the years and share it with others. I decided to dedicate my career, and my life, to helping others suffering from AF. In this book, I will share the things I do to have fewer bouts of AF. I will share the insights developed from watching countless procedures, and from the hours of conversations I have had with physicians strategizing on the best way to approach each individual patient based on their needs and situation. My hope is that these insights can help you reduce your risk of stroke and possibly eliminate your AF altogether.

You are likely frightened and anxious and feel isolated. Most of all, you want to get answers. In the chapters that follow, I'll explain AF and how it relates to stroke. I'll share my insights about the types of doctors available to help treat AF, so you can find the best doctor for YOU.

And, I'll explain the medical treatments available so that you can make an informed decision about the treatment that is best for your unique situation. I'll also explain how to eliminate bad foods from your diet, and incorporate healthy ones. Finally, I'll give you an easy, step-by-step plan to add exercise to your daily routine and give you proven methods for handling and eliminating stress.

AF can occur at any time. It may be related to factors that can be controlled, or to factors that cannot, like age or heredity. Once you experience AF, it is likely you will experience it repeatedly. There is no cookie cutter approach to dealing with AF. Your AF is unique to you. It will arrive unexpectedly and stay for as long as it wants. Because each situation is unique, my objective is to offer all the information in one place to assist you in making the decisions that could help improve your life.

Because I suffer from and live with AF, I have done the research necessary to increase my knowledge. The difference between you searching, and me searching, is that I know what I'm looking for. The information is out there, but it seems scattered in dozens of different places. And, some of the information may seem decent until you look at the small print and see it is written or sponsored by a pharmaceutical or device company. Obviously, these companies are trying to sell medication and a closer look reveals the information is slanted to take you down their road of treatment. This is flat out biased and may not be immediately obvious to the typical consumer.

Again, I thought of you. When you are frightened, lonely, fearful of death, and in need of answers—do you really have the time or energy to sit at the computer wandering aimlessly to find straightforward information? I don't think so; and that is another reason why I wrote this book, as a source you can turn to for the essential information you need to beat AF and reduce your risk of stroke.

I want you to know—I get it. I know how you feel, and I want to help you.

It is vitally important to understand how AF can affect your life. Most of all, you need to know what you can do to control your AF. It can weigh on your mind and cause excessive stress, which is a major trigger for AF. It is critical to gain control over your AF by understanding how to self-manage the areas of your life that you can control; and make decisions in order to seek help in areas of your life that seem out of control. When you begin to recognize what contributes to this condition, it will be easier for you to deal with it and make a plan to overcome it. My goal is to provide pathways to make this possible for you. Reading this book will put you on a path toward achieving a happy, healthy lifestyle; with a renewed spirit and a heart in normal rhythm.

Open your mind and give yourself the chance to make changes to your lifestyle. Consider and follow the advice I am sharing with you in this book. You will be empowered to take action and witness improvements in your health. If you don't act, your life may continue to spiral out of control.

I believe in you. I admire your goal to learn about AF and take control of your future. My purpose: make your battle become easier by sharing all I know. You can start improving your heart health right away.

Chapter 1

Understand AF and Your Risk of Stroke

"Healing is a matter of time, but it is also sometimes a matter of opportunity."

- Hippocrates

Atrial fibrillation is the most common type of irregular
heartbeat. This irregular heartbeat is called an arrhythmia, which means your heart beats in an abnormal rhythm.
A common experience many of us may have had is a racing
heart after too much caffeine. Often, after that super high-
test coffee or energy drink, our normal heartbeat becomes
very fast and irregular. This is similar to how AF feels.

Your heart is electrically-charged. It is designed to efficiently pump blood throughout your body. The top of your
heart (atria) and the bottom of your heart (ventricles) are
designed to work in unison. If the top of your heart produces
chaotic electrical signals, your heart begins to fibrillate or
quiver.

This causes the bottom of your heart to begin quivering
as it tries to continue working in unison with the top. The
result is an irregular rapid beat known as AF.

AF Impacts Millions of People

Atrial fibrillation affects approximately 10 million people in the US and Europe, and 33.5 million people worldwide.[1]

Some medical researchers believe that only one-third of those with AF actually know they have it.

Once you reach the age of 40, you have a 1 in 4 chance of developing AF. It affects women, men, and children, both athletes and those with more sedentary lifestyles. AF is the most common heart condition. It can impact anyone, in any social class, in any country, in any walk of life. By 2050, it is expected that in the United States alone, as many as 15.9 million people will suffer from AF.[2] It seems to me this is becoming an epidemic, and I want to do something to help stop its progression.

My purpose is to provide awareness and information to help you understand this dangerous condition. In this book, I will outline the many techniques you can use to naturally manage the symptoms and underlying causes that aggravate AF. And most of all, I want to steer you toward understanding the ways this condition can be treated and ultimately decrease your risk of stroke, which is the biggest risk factor of this disease.

Risk of Stroke Increases with AF

Atrial fibrillation increases your risk of stroke by as much as five times.[3] A stroke is when the blood supply to your brain is stopped or slowed due to a blockage (clot).

---

[1] Chugh, et al. "Worldwide Epidemiology of Atrial Fibrillation." Circulation, 129: 837-847 (2014).

[2] Physiciansweekly.com, August 29, 2012. November 11, 2016. <physiciansweekly.com/atrial-fibrillation-awareness-month/>.

[3] Webmd.com, August 4, 2016. <webmd.com/heartdisease/atrialfibrillation/ss/slideshow-af-overview>.

When the brain is not being supplied with blood, its cells begin to die, and brain damage or other severe complications may result.

The reason AF so significantly increases the chance of stroke is during AF your heart is quivering and not actually pumping or ejecting the blood from your heart normally. The blood that remains in your heart can begin to form a clot. If a clot forms and leaves the heart, the effects may be extremely dangerous. Should the clot travel to the brain, for example, it will move through blood vessels until it becomes stuck. Larger clots get lodged faster because they do not fit through tiny blood vessels. If the clot is small however, it can travel quite far and become lodged in a very tiny vessel. Where the clot lodges and constricts blood flow affects the stroke's consequences, which may include numbness, weakness, stiffness, and the inability to speak, to form thoughts, to remember facts, names, or how to perform everyday actions, such as walking or eating. A stroke can be so debilitating that you need 24-hour care. Or worse, a stroke may be caused by a clot so large that much of your brain is deprived of oxygen, resulting in death. In addition to stroke, over time, AF can weaken the strength of your heart and lead to heart failure, which can also lead to death.

Atrial fibrillation is linked to approximately 15% of the strokes in the US alone.[3] As patients with AF age, their chances of having a stroke increase. Unfortunately, AF-related strokes are usually twice as likely to be deadly or extremely debilitating compared to non-AF strokes.

Sadly, about half of all who suffer from a stroke linked to AF will die within a year. Stroke is the most common fear

---

[3] Warner, Jennifer. WebMD.com. March 7, 2011. November 7, 2016. <webmd.com/heart-disease/atrialfibrillation/news/20110307/atrial-fibrillation4737026996429004-may-have-link-to-dimentia?print=true>.

and complication related to AF, but the good news is—many of these strokes can be prevented with proper treatment, which I will discuss in Chapter 5.

How to Determine Your Risk of Stroke

The most common way to determine your risk of stroke is to use an assessment calculator called the CHADS-VASc scoring criteria. Each letter stands for a complication that puts you at an increased risk for having a stroke. This tool is widely accepted and used by the medical community to assess the risk. According to the Heart Rhythm Society (an international organization that promotes education related to arrhythmias for both patients and professionals), a score of "0" is associated with a low risk of stroke (possibly requiring aspirin), a score of "1" relates to an intermediate risk (requiring at least aspirin) and any score higher than 1 is considered a high risk requiring some type of therapy.

In the chart to the right, there is a description (in the middle column) of each letter in the CHADS-VASc calculator. For example, C stands for Congestive Heart Failure, H stands for Hypertension, and so on through the letters. If you are comfortable with determining whether or not you have the conditions listed in middle column, this is a simple tool to determine your risk. If you are not comfortable or do not know enough about your health history, you can ask your doctor to help you use the CHADS-VASc scoring system to determine your risk. In either case, the score determines the treatment you need which ultimately should be discussed with your doctor.

To begin, ask yourself – "Do I have congestive heart failure?" If you are certain based on a diagnosis from your doctor that you do, check the box and give yourself 1 point. If you know you do not have congestive heart failure, leave the box empty and move on to the next condition. The next question is "do you suffer from hypertension?" If yes, 1 point is given, if not move on to the next condition. You will continue through the exercise and tally your score at the end adding up the points for any condition you check off. You will notice some categories are worth 2 points. For example, if you have had a prior stroke, you would give yourself 2 points. The same is true if you are over 75. Once you determine your score, share the results with your doctor and he or she can work with you to formulate a therapy plan.

Check box if this risk applies	Description of Risk Factor	# of points assigned
	Congestive Heart Failure	1
	Hypertension	1
	Age - Older than 75?	2
	Diabetes Millitus	1
	Stroke, TIA, or thromboembolism	2
	Vascular Disease, previous MI, peripheral artery disease or aortic plaque	1
	Age 65-74	1
	Gender is female	1

TOTAL SCORE _____

The Three Types of AF

Atrial fibrillation is typically considered a progressive disease that includes three types or classifications. Atrial fibrillation often starts by occurring with brief episodes. However, in some cases AF can start at a more severe or continuous level. No matter what stage it begins, the longer atrial fibrillation is left untreated or not controlled, the harder it can become to treat.

The most common type is called **Paroxysmal AF**. It is usually very symptomatic, which means you feel your heart racing or thumping and can easily recognize that it is beating irregularly. AF, in this stage, can last for as long as seven days or for as little as several hours, minutes or a few seconds at a time. During paroxysmal AF, the heart goes in and out of normal rhythm, but eventually returns to normal on its own. The majority of people with AF (approximately two out of three) have paroxysmal AF and don't even realize it.

Persistent AF lasts more than seven days and requires medical assistance to force the heart back into normal rhythm. If you have persistent AF, a medical professional will usually administer medication to help the heart return to normal. If this doesn't work, you may require cardioversion (electrical shock). If you ignore persistent AF, or refuse appropriate treatment, and it lasts more than a year, the condition is then called **long-standing persistent AF**.

Permanent AF occurs when your heart is always beating irregularly. Patients with permanent AF can be much less responsive to medication, most procedures, and even cardioversion. In some cases, a heart in permanent AF will never return to normal rhythm.

The Left Atrial Appendage

So, where, exactly, does a clot usually form? During the third week of embryonic development, the left atrium of the heart forms. As the heart continues to develop, a leftover sac or attachment, referred to as the left atrial appendage, develops. This sac is located on the left side of the upper part of your left atrium and is believed to be the place where 90% of the clots that cause stroke are formed.

For this reason, this structure has been called the lethal attachment. It is the silent killer for those with AF because it is impossible to feel the clot forming in the left atrial appendage. Blood has a natural tendency to clot and this sac is a place where blood can easily gather, congeal, and clot, thereby greatly increasing the risk for stroke.

Chapter 2

Recognize the Symptoms of AF

"Many admire, few know."

- Hippocrates

I have a friend in his early 60's who is overweight and has a stressful job. He does not maintain a healthy sleep schedule or lifestyle, and I have warned him that he is a ticking time bomb for AF, or other heart disease. One Friday morning, he woke and felt horrible. His chest was pounding, his heart was racing and fluttering out of control, he was out of breath, and could hardly make it to the bathroom without falling over. He thought he was having a heart attack. The night before he went to dinner with clients (which no doubt included the customary salty food served in many restaurants), he had a few cocktails and wine with dinner, barely drank any water, got home late and, not surprisingly, had a lousy night's sleep. I told him that he basically created the perfect storm, and what he experienced that Friday morning was likely AF. It was enough to scare him, and fortunately he has made drastic changes to his life.

If you are reading this book, you may already know or suspect you have AF. You may already be aware of some or many of the symptoms, or you may have recently been diagnosed and were not aware that you had it, or the symptoms may have gone unnoticed. AF can be symptomatic, meaning you know as soon as the heart begins to fibrillate or quiver. Or, surprisingly, for approximately two thirds of all sufferers, it can be asymptomatic, meaning you may have this condition and do not realize it. As I mentioned earlier, when you have Paroxysmal AF, you are usually symptomatic and acutely aware of your irregular heartbeat. As the disease progresses, you may become used to the irregular beat and accustomed to simply not feeling healthy.

Common Symptoms

Regardless of the AF stage you are in, at some point, you will likely experience one or more of these symptoms:

Anxiety

Chest pressure or chest pain
(which may require medical attention)

Chest tightness or discomfort

Dizziness or lightheadedness

Faintness or confusion

Restless or feeling unsettled and unable to calm down

Feeling tired or having a lack of energy

Fluttering or thumping in the chest

Increased urination

Rapid or irregular heartbeat

Shortness of breath

Chapter 3

Identify Common Causes and Triggers

"It is more important to know what sort of person
has a disease, than to know what sort of disease
the person has."

- Hippocrates

There are many causes of AF. Each person has individual reasons why this condition has taken hold. The list below contains common causes; however, AF is complicated and your AF may be a result of multiple factors and causes. In rare cases, AF cannot be explained and a reason can be difficult to pinpoint.

Age - there is a 25% chance of developing AF once you turn 40

Alcohol - even in moderate use, alcohol can trigger and cause AF

Anxiety - any activity that causes over-production of adrenalin or cortisol, such as fear; or even a stressful conversation or event

Caffeine - increases blood pressure and heart rate, is linked to AF

Cardiomyopathy - weakened heart muscle

Cigarettes/Nicotine - increases heart rate, blood pressure, and causes AF

Coronary artery disease - plaque builds up in the arteries of the heart, which blocks oxygen-rich blood from reaching all parts of the heart

Dehydration - an excessive loss of water

Diabetes - the inability of the body to produce adequate insulin, which causes high glucose levels in the blood

Emphysema - occurs when air sacs in the lungs are damaged and cause breathlessness

Electrolyte imbalance - occurs when electrically charged particles (sodium, potassium, calcium, and magnesium) that help your heart beat become higher or lower than normal

Exhaustion - sleep deprivation

Extreme exercise and years of endurance training - marathon, rowing, triathlon, swimming, biking, or any sport where your heart rate remains elevated for extended periods of time

Genetic factors - such as age, gender or possibly family history

Heart Attack - AF can occur during a heart attack

Heart birth defects - abnormal formation of the heart before birth

Heart failure - failure for the heart to pump blood efficiently

Heart surgery - 20-30% suffer AF after heart surgery

Heart valve diseases - occur when the valves fail to open or close, making the heart lose the ability to pump blood efficiently

High blood pressure - occurs when the blood in the vessels is at a higher than normal pressure

High doses of steroids or NSAIDS - or other over the counter stimulant drugs

Hyperthyroidism - over-activity of the thyroid gland, which results in a rapid heart rate

Illegal stimulant drugs - include any drug taken with a non-medical purpose in mind

Lung disease - any problem in the lungs that causes narrowing or blockage of the airway

Obesity - excessive storage of fat in the body resulting in a weight that is considered unhealthy for a given height

Pericarditis - inflammation of the sac that holds your heart

Poor diet - eating processed foods high in sodium and sugar instead of whole foods with necessary nutrients

Rheumatic fever/heart disease - inflammation of the heart muscle or scarring of the valves of the heart

Sedentary lifestyle - lack of proper movement and exercise

Sick sinus syndrome - electrical misfires occurring that cause the heart to speed up or slow down

Sleep apnea - a sleep disorder characterized by shallow breathing or long pauses in your breathing, which can last from a few seconds to minutes

Stress - an emotionally, physically, or mentally challenging circumstance that causes a hormonal reaction or chemical response by the body

In my own experience, the biggest problem is when multiple triggers or causes are occurring at or near the same time together. In other words, if I am exhausted, dehydrated and have a glass or two of wine, it is more likely that I will experience AF. I have learned that I cannot allow multiple causes, triggers or factors to work together or else I face a higher immediate risk for AF.

Take a close look at your day. Look to decrease your exposure to the things that might trigger AF. This can be a challenging process, but you can accomplish it with a strong will and motivation. If you make it a goal to change just one thing each week, it won't be long before you have a grip on everything that may be contributing to your AF.

Chapter 4

Choose the Right Doctor

"Wherever the art of medicine is loved,
there is also a love of humanity."

– Hippocrates

Doctors with differing training and experience may play important roles in the diagnosis and treatment of AF. This chapter offers descriptions of the various categories of doctors that have the ability to help you with your AF.

General Practitioner (GP)/family doctor/primary care doctor

A GP, family doctor or primary care doctor, is a non-specialized medical doctor. Depending on your country of origin, the role of this doctor can vary. For example, in rural sections of some countries a General Practitioner, family doctor or primary care doctor may be very involved in the care of patients and have the liberty to treat more complex health issues. In other countries, these doctors are less involved in extensive treatments of major health issues and more quickly refer your care to a specialist.

In most cases, a GP or family doctor should be able to detect AF. If a GP or family doctor discovers you have AF, it is often at an early stage, typically during a routine or regular check-up (which is why it is recommended you see your doctor once a year for an annual physical). GPs and family doctors treat both genders and generally see patients of any age. They can treat many illnesses, but in the case of AF, they will likely refer you to a specialized physician.

Cardiologist

A cardiologist can diagnose, treat and help prevent diseases of the heart and blood vessels. They treat heart attacks, heart failure, as well as heart rhythm disorders.

Cardiologists often perform stress tests, echocardiograms (ultrasounds of the heart to diagnose disease), and ambulatory echocardiograms (record electrical activity of your heart while you are performing an activity), as well as interpret the results of these tests. Cardiologists are not all trained to perform invasive medical procedures, such as cardiac catheterizations (procedures done to diagnose or treat conditions of the heart by inserting a long thin tube called a catheter through blood vessels in the groin, neck or arm and into the heart). However, all cardiologists are able to prescribe medications that treat AF, such as heart rate control or rhythm control drugs.

Electrophysiologist

An electrophysiologist, or EP, is a cardiologist with specialized training in heart rhythm disorders and the electrical system of the heart. An EP's training focuses on the study of electrical properties of the heart-related biological cells and tissue. Only about 5% of cardiologists specialize to become electrophysiologists.

EPs can also perform the same tests as cardiologists, prescribe medication, and perform invasive procedures including cardiac ablation (freezing or heating the heart tissue that is producing chaotic electrical signals and causing AF).

Cardiac or Cardiovascular Surgeon

Cardiac or Cardiovascular surgeons have extensive education and training in performing specialized procedures within the human chest, primarily on the heart. They perform the following:

— aneurysm repair (blood vessels that have bulged and are in danger of bursting) of the large arteries in the chest

— cardiac ablation for the treatment of AF

— coronary artery bypass surgery

— heart transplants

— ligation of the left atrial appendage (a surgical procedure to close the left atrial appendage and prevent blood from entering this attachment, where most clots form)

— operations on blockages or leaks in the heart or its vessels

— treatment for heart failure

— treatments for congenital heart conditions (problems with the heart that occur during fetal development)

— valve replacements or valve repairs

plus any other procedure to treat damage caused by diseases or disorders of the cardiovascular system.

In many cases, these highly skilled surgeons can also treat disorders associated with the lungs, esophagus or chest wall.

Chapter 5

Know Your Medical Treatment Options

**"Extreme remedies are very appropriate
for extreme diseases."**

- Hippocrates

The chart below is a great visual tool to understand the various paths of treatment typically offered by the doctors you see. Each treatment will be described in detail later in this chapter.

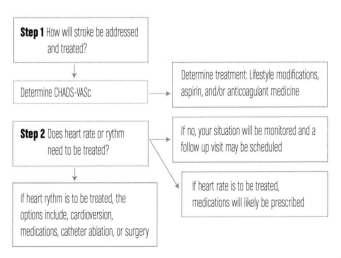

The best treatment for your AF is usually determined through consideration of a variety of factors including how long you have been experiencing AF, whether or not you have other structural heart issues, other medical problems you may be facing, and the overall severity of your heart arrhythmia. Depending on your age and lifestyle, you may want to seek multiple opinions before you decide what path to take for your treatment. For example, you may have to decide if you want to use medication to treat your AF, which in many cases can be very successful, or have a procedure that can possibly put your heart back into normal rhythm without medication. Your initial treatment may depend on what type of doctor you see first, as some doctors are trained to perform corrective procedures and others are not. The latter may prescribe drugs as your first mode of treatment or refer your care to another type of physician if the drugs do not work or your case is more severe.

For the ease of definition and to help you decipher the types of treatment, I will simply define each of the terms below. For all medications, the generic names are listed. If medication is prescribed, ask your physician for the generic name of the drug(s) prescribed, as your doctor may prescribe a brand name rather than a generic version of the medication. Doing so will enable you to do research and obtain information about the drug you are taking. After the overview of medications, we will take a look at the medical procedures used to correct AF.

AF Treatment Medications

As you know, having AF brings a significantly-increased risk of stroke. The common goal of any AF treatment is to manage the condition in a way that dramatically reduces or eliminates the risk of stroke, and helps your heartbeat return to normal.

The first course of treatment is usually medication. Medications include blood thinners, rate control and rhythm control drugs. Drugs do not cure AF; they simply suppress it, manage the symptoms that are difficult to live with, and decrease the factors that put you at risk for stroke. Prior to determining the type of medication, your doctor will likely perform an echocardiogram, stress test, check to see if you suffer from cardiomyopathy (disease in the heart muscle), as well as other types of diagnosis to assess your situation.

Anticoagulation medication (blood thinners)

This drug class is often prescribed to prevent and treat blood clot formation. Aspirin is a blood-thinning agent, but has not been proven to reduce the risk of stroke. However, aspirin is the first course of action recommended by the Heart Rhythm Society for patients with a CHADS-VASc score of zero or one. Other common drugs in this category are warfarin (which requires monthly testing to make sure you are receiving the optimal dose), dabigatran, rivaroxaban, and apixaban.

Most of these drugs carry an increased risk of bleeding (and bruising) since they are intended to thin your blood and take away its ability to clot.

Before taking anti-clotting medication, tell your doctor about all other types of medications or supplements you are taking, or special dietary restrictions you may have. These factors can change the effect anti-clotting medication can have on your body.

You should also tell your pharmacist and all other doctors you may consult, including your dentist, that you are taking blood thinners. It is very important, especially if you need a procedure that can cause bleeding or where your inability to clot could become a dangerous factor.

These drugs are prescribed with strict guidelines. If you forget to take a dose, you should not take an extra dose. This is quite dangerous. If bleeding or bruising becomes an issue, immediately contact your healthcare provider. These symptoms can be life-threatening. Other circumstances or conditions that may require medical attention when taking these medications include an accident or fall; faintness, weakness or dizziness; red, dark brown or black stools or urine; excessive bleeding with your period; stomachaches or headaches that will not subside; or bleeding gums. Many of these drugs have a long list of other side effects, dangers, and variables you should be aware of before taking them. Do your homework and look up anything you have been prescribed, so that you are well informed about the medications going into your body.

Rate Control Drugs

In order to manage your heart rate, the frequency or speed at which your heart is beating, your physician may prescribe a rate control drug. These drugs are designed to keep your heart rate within the normal range. Often, these drugs provide immediate relief, as they tend to slow the rate so that you don't feel like your heart is constantly pounding.

Beta blockers are a type of rate control drug and include timolol, propranolol, atenolol, bisoprolol, metoprolol, and carvedilol. Calcium channel blockers are another rate control medication, which not only slow the rate, but also reduce the strength of the muscles' cell contractions so that your heart won't be able to beat so quickly. Examples of calcium channel blockers are verapamil and diltiazem. The last medication that falls into this category is digoxin, which regulates the electrical currents being conducted to the bottom part of your heart from the top part of your heart.

Rhythm Control Drugs

Once the rate is controlled and the heart is beating at a normal speed, physicians usually then try to control the rhythm. A rhythm control drug regulates the tempo, pace, or cadence of your heart. In other words, it regulates your pulse and keeps it constant and within the normal range.

The first types of rhythm control drugs are sodium channel blockers. Common examples of sodium channel blockers include flecainide, and propafenone. All of these drugs slow down the ability of your heart to produce electricity. Another type, potassium channel blockers, actually slows down the electrical signals that cause AF.

A few examples are amiodarone, sotalol, and dofetilide.

Once again, while drugs can provide relief to your heart and help regulate it, they are not a cure for AF. Their overall success rates vary greatly and each medication may have a long list of side effects. In addition, drug therapy typically requires close monitoring and frequent doctor visits. The requirements associated with monitoring sometimes cause patients to stop taking their medication, which also carries a risk.

Procedures for Treating AF

If you, in consultation with your doctor, decide the pharmaceutical approach is not effective, or does not fit your lifestyle, there are several types of procedures that may be appropriately performed in an attempt to terminate your AF.

Catheter Ablation

Catheter ablations are performed by an electrophysiologist. During this procedure, a series of thin flexible wires are guided into a blood vessel, usually located in your groin. The catheters are then steered up into your heart. The first step is to locate the areas of your heart that are producing the chaotic signals responsible for the AF. Next, the special electrodes located at the end of the catheter are sent energy from a machine. This energy is delivered in the form of radiofrequency or cryotherapeutic energy and is intended to burn (radiofrequency) or freeze (cryotherapy) the tissue. The electrophysiologist will likely do a series of burns (or freezes), and the extent of what they perform is based on your individual situation. The success rate for catheter ablation ranges between 53.1% and 79.8%.[1] In cases where large areas of the atria are destroyed during this procedure, a pacemaker may be needed to make the heart contract in a normal manner.

Surgical Ablation Techniques

Surgical treatments are usually offered to patients with AF who did not have success with medication, had unsuccessful catheter ablation(s), have an enlarged left atrium or blood clots in the left atrium, have a history of stroke, or have other heart problems that require surgical intervention. There are risks associated with cardiac surgery that include infections, damage to heart tissue, kidneys, liver or lungs, memory loss, etc. Your doctor will discuss what risks you may face, since those are determined on an individual basis.

The **Cox-Maze IV** is a more advanced surgical procedure most commonly done to comprehensively treat AF. It consists of a series of cuts and burns or freezes made to kill tissue and interrupt the electrical pathways causing your AF. Cox-Maze IV creates a series of lesions on both the right and left atrium. The lesions or incisions ultimately create scars that run the width of the heart muscle and inhibit

[1] Ganesan, Shipp, Brooks, et al. "Long-term Outcomes of Catheter Ablation of Atrial Fibrillation: A Systematic Review and Meta-analysis." Journal of American Heart Association. 2013; 2:e004549.

the faulty signals from traveling through the (now scarred) heart muscle. The technology used for this procedure is radiofrequency and/or cryotherapy. Radiofrequency energy kills the faulty tissue through the heating of the cells in the heart muscle, and cryotherapy freezes the tissue to a state where the cells will not survive and no longer conduct the poor electrical signals that cause AF.

Surgical ablation can be performed during open chest surgery or through small openings made between your ribs. Typically, if you have AF and other heart problems that require surgery, such as coronary artery disease or valve disease, your surgeon will likely repair all of your ailments during the same procedure. The success rate of the Cox-Maze IV procedure is approximately 80%, which includes patients at all levels of severity.[2]

The Society of Thoracic Surgeons (STS) is the governing body for the cardiac surgery community in the United States, which is comprised of 7,400 surgeons who are dedicated to the best possible surgical care for heart, lung, esophagus and other organs in the chest. In December of 2016, the STS released new guidelines for the surgical treatment of atrial fibrillation. They have determined that it is recommended to perform surgical ablation on all patients who have atrial fibrillation during the time they are getting structural heart surgery. They now believe this surgery is not only safe and effective, but believe it should be done. Similar to STS, the AATS (American Association for Thoracic Surgery) and HRS (Heart Rhythm Society) have also modified their guidelines and now support ablation for patients with atrial fibrillation. Now, all three major societies in the U.S. (and

---

[2] Michael O'Riordan. "Two-thirds of Patients Free from AF Without Drugs 5 Years After Surgical Ablation." <Medscape.com/viewarticle/849694>.

most European Societies) support and recommend concomitant, surgical, catheter and/or hybrid ablation for patients with atrial fibrillation. The support of these groups is considered monumental and further substantiates the need to medically address a condition impacting more and more people worldwide.

If you only have AF, and do not have other heart disease, there is a minimally invasive procedure called the TT, Totally Thoracoscopic, or VATS (Video-Assisted Thoracoscopic Surgery) maze that can be done. These procedures are usually done through small openings made between the ribs. The surgeon will typically use radiofrequency to burn the tissue during these minimally invasive procedures.

During surgical maze procedures, it is assumed that the left atrial appendage will be cut off, removed, or excluded in some fashion. As 90% of clots that cause stroke originate from the left atrial appendage, this procedure includes its removal. If the appendage is gone, a clot cannot form in it!

The left atrial appendage can be treated a few ways. A surgeon may excise (cut off) the appendage and sew the opening closed with stitches. Other methods include implanting a device during cardiac surgery, which is intended to exclude the left atrial appendage.

Other devices are implanted by electrophysiologists. These products are guided through a catheter, through the groin and placed at the opening of the left atrial appendage from inside of the heart.

As with any procedure, you can ask your physician the following types of questions: how do they treat the left atrial appendage, what device or approach do they use to close off the appendage, ask about the FDA approval associated with the device or method used, ask how many times the device discussed has been implanted, ask about the success rate of the device or method discussed, and ask for a copy of the research or literature supporting the method or device discussed. It is also suggested the information shared is confirmed by further researching the device and complication rates on-line or with other doctors. Be an informed patient and do your homework. Remember it is your treatment, and if your doctor doesn't want to use the device or approach you think is best for you or you are not satisfied with your doctor's reasoning, then there is always the option to seek another opinion.

In the end, it is important that you have the left atrial appendage treated on its own or as a part of a surgical procedure. Your life can drastically improve knowing that the place where most clots form has been properly treated.

Hybrid Ablation

Another method for treating patients with AF is a hybrid ablation. This is a combined approach, which utilizes the skills of both the electrophysiologist and the cardiac surgeon. Typically, the patients who qualify for this approach have had at least one catheter ablation, but still suffer from AF, and have no other structural heart disease. The technology most commonly used in this method is radiofrequency ablation performed on the outside of the heart muscle by the cardiac surgeon, and radiofrequency or cryotherapy delivered through the catheter to the inside of the heart by the electrophysiologist. This procedure is usually done in a staged manner, with the surgical procedure first followed, the next day or even months later, by the catheter-based approach. This method of ablation is gaining in popularity and success ranges from 75-90+% depending on the team of doctors and the combination of technologies used.

Ask your doctor about his or her approach, what devices will be used, how many procedures he or she has done, and their success rate. This information is easy to confirm with a little bit of online research, which you should review and evaluate. Also, the FDA is highly involved in the approval of the products available on the market used to treat AF, as well as the left atrial appendage. Its website is a source of valuable information. Getting multiple opinions prior to making a decision is also a useful strategy.

Once you have a procedure, whether catheter, surgical, or hybrid, it is widely acceptable to consider whether it was successful after 90 days. This waiting period is needed for the scars and lesions to fully mature and form, further creating the block needed to interrupt the bad electrical signals from traveling across your heart.

Chapter 6

Eat Right for a Healthy Heart

"Let food be thy medicine and
medicine be thy food."

- Hippocrates

If you already have AF, your diet will not reverse the arrhythmia. However, diet plays a vital role in how you feel, and can influence how your heart health progresses. In this chapter, I will outline the foods to avoid, and the foods you should include in your meals, for the rest of your life. I have dramatically changed what and how I eat over the past five years, and truly believe I am healthier than ever. I have no plans of reverting because I experience fewer bouts of AF since making these healthy changes.

I do not like to focus on the word diet. To me, diet sounds temporary, like a phase used to accomplish a short-term goal. I view the food that I put into my mouth as fuel for my system and nourishment for my body. I look at my heart and body as a gift that I am now trying to preserve. Once you have this mindset, you will no longer see food and drink as anything else. In the majority of cases, food has been found to play a major role in contributing to AF. Why continue to pollute your system? I want to help you to make positive changes and offer ways to improve what and how you eat.

The foundation of eating properly includes foods that are rich in vitamins and minerals. Making sure you eat these kinds of foods guarantees you are filling your body with the macro and micronutrients on which your system depends for survival. Having the right balance of vitamins and minerals enhances your overall health. On the contrary, a diet with prolonged deficiencies can lead to extreme health problems impacting more than just your heart. It is also best to get your vitamins and minerals from food, and not rely on supplements, since high doses of any mineral or vitamin can produce toxic reactions.

Whole foods, like the ones listed in this section, are complex; they contain many vitamins and minerals. Whole foods are also rich in fiber, which can prevent disease and aid in digestion. Whole foods also contain phytochemicals, which can protect against diabetes and heart disease. If you rely on supplements, you miss the beneficial, naturally occurring chemicals found in whole foods. Proper combinations of whole foods, in the form of vegetables, fruits, beans, and grains, work together to give your body exactly what it needs to function properly and maintain good health.

There are some cases where supplements may be beneficial. Discuss with your doctor if supplements are necessary for you. For example, if you are postmenopausal, over the age of 50, eat a diet lacking proper calories (2,000 per day on average), are vegan or vegetarian, have digestive problems, smoke, are pregnant, or drink in excess, you may benefit from supplements.

Here is a list of the average number of milligrams of essential vitamins and minerals needed each day:

- Biotin 300 mcg
- Calcium 1,000-1,200 mg
- Chloride 3,400 mg
- Chromium 120 mcg
- Copper 2 mg
- Iodine 150 mcg
- Iron 18 mg
- Magnesium 400 mg for men/320 mg for women
- Manganese 2 mg
- Molybdenum 75 mcg
- Pantothenic acid 10 mg
- Phosphorus 1,000 mg
- Potassium 3,500 - 4,700 mg
- Selenium 70 mcg
- Sodium 2,400 mg
- Vitamin A 5,000 IU
- Vitamin B-1 (thiamin) 1.5 mg
- Vitamin B-2 (riboflavin) 1.7 mg
- Vitamin B-3 (niacin) 20 mg
- Vitamin B-6 2 mg
- Vitamin B-9 (folic acid) 400 mcg
- Vitamin B-12 6 mcg
- Vitamin C 60 mg
- Vitamin D 400 IU
- Vitamin E 30 IU

- Vitamin K 80 mcg
- Zinc 15 mg

Eliminating Bad Foods from Your Diet

The first step to eating for a healthy heart is to remove from your cabinets and refrigerator any unhealthy foods that may trigger your AF. Don't leave any of the following items around since they will likely tempt you, take you backward on your journey, and possibly lead to more bouts of AF.

The Worst Foods for Heart Health and AF:

- **Alcohol** - Wine, beer and hard alcohols are a trigger, and over-indulgence in any type of alcohol is problematic. If you can, stop drinking entirely. If you cannot, seek help.

- **Fried foods** - such as chicken, French fries, potato chips (or any chips in a bag)

- **Iodized table salt** - All iodized table salt in your home should be replaced with Himalayan sea salt. Salt provides sodium and chloride, which are both needed (and not created) by your body. However, you only need about 1,500 mg of sodium a day. You do not need the excessive amount in white table salt. Natural salt, such as Himalayan sea salt, contains 84% sodium chloride (37% of which is pure sodium). The remaining 16% is made up of trace minerals. Himalayan sea salt is pink in color and has almost 0.3% potassium, which is a vital mineral your body also needs. Table salt, on the other hand, contains almost 98% sodium chloride (39% of which is pure sodium). The remainder in table salt is made up of man-made chemicals that have no business being in your body. In addition to Himalayan sea salt, Celtic salt is another great alternative. Celtic sea salt is grey or almost light purple in color, harvested from coastal areas in France, and carries many of the same benefits of Himalayan sea salt.

- **Processed breakfast foods** - such as donuts, muffins, bagels, or danish
- **Processed foods high in salt** - read the sodium content and compare before you buy
- **Processed meats** - lunch meats, hot dogs, sausage or any meat that does not come from grass-fed animals
- **Soda and energy drinks** - There is nothing healthy or valuable in soda or energy drinks. And, "diet" soda is not healthier. All soda has either dangerously high levels of sugar or dangerous artificial sweeteners (used in diet soda). Most soda and energy drinks contain caffeine, which is linked to a host of other problems including irregular heartbeat and high blood pressure. Eliminate these immediately.
- **Sugar** - If you must, opt for natural sugar, not the white sugars sold in pound bags. An alternative natural sugar to use is coconut sugar. Coconut sugar comes from the sap of the coconut palm tree. Unlike regular sugar, coconut sugar has valuable minerals such as iron, zinc, calcium and potassium. The glycemic value is also much lower than table sugar, it raises your blood sugar level much more slowly, and has a fiber called inulin, which has been found to slow glucose absorption. I use Coconut Secret Raw Coconut Crystals, which can be bought online or at your local grocery store.
- **Sweetened dairy** - such as ice cream, low fat ice cream, or frozen yogurt
- **Trans fats and saturated trans fats** - such as margarine, and those found in baked goods and fast food

- **White flour or any gluten products** - refined grains, white rice, crackers, and white pasta

Regardless of how often you experience AF, proper food choices will help reduce your risk as well as reduce your symptoms. Begin making smart choices and get yourself on the road to better health. Even if AF were not an issue in your life, the above changes will improve overall health for anyone. It is because these food items have become so ingrained in our society that AF and many other types of disease are on the rise.

Limit Your Calories

In addition to eliminating foods that are not good for you or your condition, you should limit your daily caloric intake to the recommended amount of 2,000 calories. Being overweight contributes to many risk factors that worsen your symptoms. A heart-healthy diet is an aspect of your life you can control. The choices you make at the grocery store, in restaurants, and in your kitchen each day will start making you feel healthier. It is not so much any one meal, or the one or two times a week you decide to "live a little," but when you make bad choices every day, for weeks, then years, your body will be unable to safely process and dispose of the impurities. All too often, the result is obesity, poor heart health, and other lifethreatening conditions. Enjoying a wonderful, indulgent meal, once in a while, is fine. But using your will power and mental strength to do what is best for your body on a regular basis will keep your heart ticking at its best for years to come. Whole, unprocessed foods were naturally put on this earth as a source of fuel for our bodies. Food is meant to help us maintain the energy and nutrients we need to go about our life. You can think of your stomach as your fuel tank. In the same way you wouldn't put anything other than gas in your car, you shouldn't put things in your stomach that won't optimally power your body.

Foods that Fuel a Healthy Heart

Now that you know what to eliminate, I want to help you understand what you should eat and stock in your refrigerator and pantry accordingly.

The Best Foods for Heart Health and AF include:

- Apricots
- Artichokes
- Asparagus
- Avocados
- Bananas
- Beans - kidney, string, lentils; but not baked beans from a can, which are high in salt and sugar!
- Berries - any and all types
- Cantaloupe
- Cashews
- Figs
- Fish
- Garlic
- Green, leafy vegetables such as kale, spinach, lettuce, mustard greens, collard greens
- Lean grass-fed beef, lamb, bison, or poultry
- Mushrooms
- Non-leafy vegetables such as broccoli, cauliflower, Brussel sprouts, cabbage

- Nuts such as walnuts, pistachios, pine nuts, almonds (with seeds and nuts – do not buy salted. I suggest 'lightly salted with sea salt' when possible.)
- Oatmeal
- Onions
- Papaya
- Peas
- Pomegranates
- Potatoes
- Prunes
- Seeds such as flax, chia, hemp, sunflower, pumpkin, sesame
- Summer Squash
- Sweet Potatoes
- Tomatoes
- Whole Brown Rice
- Winter Squash

Whenever possible, buy fresh, organic food. These are the most desirable and beneficial foods for you and your body. You'll notice quite a few tasty choices on this list. You won't starve, you will feel satisfied; and best of all, you will be healthier and you will live longer. These foods can be eaten alone or with herbs and spices to make delicious and satisfying meals that will make your heart smile.

We have been conditioned to think of food as a source of stress relief or enjoyment. We seek the sugar-high or the satisfaction that comes from eating certain foods or drinking alcohol. The grocery store is full of items made by companies that are making millions of dollars from our bad choices. I find it motivating to buy what is best for my health, and not what is best for companies that put chemicals in food.

Although online searching for recipes with the foods or ingredients from the list above is simple, be sure to substitute proper healthy alternatives we've discussed in this chapter for the unhealthy ingredients (table salt, margarine, etc.) you may find in online recipes. For example, if you enjoy fish, simply search the internet for a delicious fish recipe.

Place the cooked fish over a bed of whole brown rice or sauteed spinach, add a side salad, and some steamed vegetables from the list. That quickly, you have a super-healthy, nutrient-rich lunch or dinner. If you love oatmeal, start your day with a bowl of oatmeal topped with fresh berries and sliced almonds.

Drink Water Daily

The last item I want to cover is water. It is vitally important to drink plenty of water. Water makes up 60% of your body weight and makes up over 70% of your heart.

Water carries nutrients from your food to your heart and other organs, and it flushes your organs and carries away waste from your body. The lifestyle of many who suffer from AF is directly linked to dehydration. I have had many people tell me, "I get my water through coffee," or, "I'm not a water drinker." However, coffee, tea and many sodas have diuretic effects and tend to dehydrate us. When we are dehydrated, the levels of electrolytes in our blood decrease to dangerous levels, which can cause abnormal heart rhythms.

It is simple to stay hydrated by eating the foods that have high water content (fruits and vegetables), and by simply drinking water throughout the day. The Institute of Medicine recommends 13 cups a day for men, which is equivalent to about 3 liters. For women, it is recommended to drink 9 cups a day, which is equivalent to approximately 2 liters of water per day.[1]

The best way to get into a habit of drinking water is to start early and drink throughout the day. In the beginning, if your body is not used to the increased water intake, you may find yourself heading to the bathroom frequently. Within a week or two this will stop. It takes some time to re-train your body that it doesn't need to survive on coffee, tea, soda, and/or alcohol. I drink water throughout the day, as often as possible, and strive to take in the recommended amount. Towards the end of the day, I stop an hour or so before bed so that I am not awakened with a full bladder at night. This system has worked well for me and I find that, as long as I'm hydrated, I have fewer incidences of AF.

---

[1] Mayo Clinic Staff. Mayoclinic.org. September 5, 2014. November 7, 2016. <mayoclinic.org/healthy-lifestyle/nutrition-an-healthy-eating/in-depth/water/art20044256>.

Chapter 7

Integrate Exercise and Reduce Stress–Easily!

*"If we could give every individual the right
amount of nourishment and exercise,
not too little and not too much, we would have
found the safest way to health."*

- Hippocrates

Before starting any exercise program, consult your physician. Experts say exercise is beneficial for people with AF, but it is important to get checked by your doctor before starting any exercise program.

Two of the biggest risk factors for stroke are high blood pressure and heart disease. Exercise is the most important physical activity you can do to reduce your blood pressure naturally for better health. I know you may feel too tired or weak to exercise. You are not alone. The majority of those who don't exercise say the same thing. But did you know that exercise actually increases energy levels over time, boosts your mood, and can improve your sex life? It does, and it can.

All it takes is 30 minutes five times a week, which is only 2.5 hours per week in total. You can start slowly, take your time, and build up to 150 minutes a week, all while making it fun and enjoyable. Gradually increasing exercise will help prevent injury and prepare your body for improved long-term health. In just a few minutes each day, you can deliver oxygen and nutrients to your cardiovascular system, release chemicals naturally in your brain that promote happiness and relaxation, sleep more soundly, improve your appearance, enhance arousal during sex for women, and decrease problems with erectile dysfunction for men. I know you want these benefits!

If you are already exercising, that is great. Keep in mind 30 minutes a day or 2.5 hours a week is a goal toward which you should progress slowly. Regardless of whether or not you are already exercising, begin each individual workout very slowly. Your heart must be warmed-up and your heart rate should not spike in the first two minutes of exercise. Do not start off with strenuous or vigorous activity. Simply start out slowly and allow your body to adapt to the new routine.

Here's how to start: This evening, before you go to bed, set your alarm a few minutes early. Begin your day with a brisk walk.

Do not plan to do it at the end of the day; by day's end, we are all tired and that becomes an easy excuse to put off the workout. If you haven't been exercising at all, start with a 5-minute walk (or an amount of time that is comfortable for you). Start slowly on your walk and increase intensity until you break a sweat or find yourself breathing a little faster. Then, the next day, walk the same amount of time, and do this five times this week. The following week, add a minute or two to each day, and continue to add a few minutes until you reach 30 minutes a day, and ultimately reach the goal of 150 minutes per week.

After each walk, drink lots of water. Then, make yourself a super-healthy breakfast. If you make this your new routine each day, you will begin to transform. This may seem like the biggest challenge of your life. Nevertheless, you can do it. It simply takes putting one foot in front of the other, and soon you will be your own success story. I can't wait for you to experience how proud of yourself you will be and how great you will feel physically and mentally. In six weeks, you will feel like a new person. It takes mere minutes a day, and those minutes will add years to your life!

Six Week Walking Plan

With this plan, you will start out slowly walking for just 5 minutes, 5 days a week and gradually build up to a heart-healthy 150 minutes per week. If you are comfortable beginning further into the following chart, feel free to do so. For example, you may be ready to jump in with 20-minute walks at the Week 4 level, and build up to 30-minute walks at the Week 6 level. The idea is to achieve the goal of 150 minutes per week, and continue doing at least this amount for the rest of your life. Vary the scenery on your walking journey. Using a treadmill is fine on rainy or cold days, but try to get outdoors and experience what nature can also do to improve your mental outlook and health. Enjoy the sites, scenes and smells of your neighborhood, a beach, or the woods! You will be amazed at what you'll discover and experience outside.

	Sun	Mon	Tues	Wed	Thurs	Fri	Sat	Total
Week 1	5 min	off	5 min	off	5 min	5 min	5 min	25 min
Week 2	8 min	off	8 min	off	8 min	8 min	8 min	40 min
Week 3	13 min	off	13 min	off	13 min	13 min	13 min	65 min
Week4	20 min	off	20 min	off	20 min	20 min	20 min	100 min
Week 5	25 min	off	25 min	off	25 min	25 min	25 min	125 min
Week 6	30 min	off	30 min	off	30 min	30 min	30 min	150 min

Tools for Managing Stress

One of the main benefits of exercise is stress relief. Exercise produces endorphins, which are the neurotransmitters in your brain that make you feel good. In addition to exercise, I have found many other ways to relax, reduce stress, calm my nerves and mind, and improve my mood and anxiety level, all of which have helped reduce my incidences of AF. Below are my favorite ways to channel my mind and energy into a positive place, even when I am in the middle of a difficult or stressful situation.

Meditate: Meditation is an excellent way to focus your attention on calming yourself and clearing your mind. This form of relaxation has been around for thousands of years and can be practiced from just a few minutes to up to 30 minutes a day.

Concentrative meditation focuses on an image, a sound, or a mantra (phrases, or words, sung, or spoken, to yourself).

Mindful meditation allows all thoughts, sounds, and images to pass through the mind freely. During mindful meditation, you are not focusing on one particular image, sound, or mantra, but rather on the free-flow of whatever positive thoughts you allow to enter your mind.

Meditation has been found to help improve the ability to deal with stress. It is a daily practice many people do at the beginning or end of the day. But it can also be used during other times, when you feel overwhelmed with stress, to regain control over your day.

Find a quiet place with minimal or no distractions. Sit on the floor or in a chair with your back straight to allow your lungs to fill with air. Close your eyes and place one hand on your belly. As you breathe in slowly say, "I love"; and as you exhale slowly, say, "Myself." Or, you can say, "I am" (as you inhale) and, "At peace" (as you exhale). Meditation takes time to master. Start out by meditating for 5 minutes and work your way up to 20 or 30 minutes a day.

Don't give up, the payoff is amazing!

Take a few deep breaths: Another way to relax and reduce stress is to focus on your breathing for 5-10 minutes. During this breathing exercise, you will sit with your back straight and shoulders back.

Close your eyes and place your hand on your belly. As you breathe in, feel your abdomen fill, then feel your chest fill, until you are full of fresh air. As you slowly exhale, be conscious of your chest, belly, and abdomen deflating and releasing all the air. Allow the bad thoughts and energy to leave your body with each exhale. And, think of your inhale as a way to pull in new and positive energy. Focus only on breathing and the power of the air you breathe and nothing else.

Focus on positive sensations: Focusing on your positive senses can be an escape and form of mental relaxation. We are constantly receiving and processing signals. We are hearing, seeing, smelling, tasting, and feeling, all at the same time. At any one moment, even during the most stressful time, our body is doing something that is worth focusing on more than the thing that is driving us crazy. For example, you can be sitting in your manager's office, or your in-law's kitchen listening to words that are causing you anxiety. If you can't escape, just tune out the negative and focus on one positive sense such as the feeling of the sun coming in the window. Gently touch your skin softly with your hand and think about how soft your skin feels, or find something in the room to glance at that is beautiful. Allow yourself to escape for a minute or two. If tuning out your audience is not possible, promise yourself a five minute walk as soon as you are able to get away. Then, during your five minutes, escape and leave the anxiety behind. Spend that time focusing on the way the air feels on your face or the smell of freshly cut grass. Simply escape and focus on one sensation that gives you joy. Live in the moment.

Make a connection: Connecting with someone is another way to release stress. If you are finding it difficult to cope with something or someone, don't let it build up inside. The stress others put on us is enough. You don't want to add to this stress by dealing with it on your own. Find someone you can confide in—pick up the phone, stop over at your neighbors, or set up a lunch date. If you are unable to find someone when you need it most, get out a journal or diary and write out everything that has you stressed, upset, angry, or unsettled. Release the negative and give your mind space to let the positive back in.

Stop stress in its tracks: We all react and carry stress differently. The problem is most of us don't realize where and how our body reacts to stress. Some people will get a rash, others will get an upset stomach, some bite their nails, others shake, and the list goes on. As soon as you find yourself getting stressed—STOP.

Immediately STOP. Do not proceed, but rather close your eyes and think about what part of your body is reacting to the stress. Focus on that part or parts of your body and work to heal it. Rather than letting the stress eat away at you, get control of your breathing, slowly count to ten and allow the fresh air coming into your lungs to make its way to the area of your body that needs the help. Imagine the air like a breeze coming in and blowing inside your body and refreshing the parts of you that are stressed.

Get a massage: A massage or tension release can work wonders. If a massage is out of the question, get a warm washcloth and place it over your eyes. If you sit, or lay down, for 10 minutes with the warm cloth, you will become relaxed. Another way to release tension is to place the warm cloth around the back of your neck. Most people get very tense in the neck and upper shoulders when they experience stress. The warmth promotes blood flow to this area, which can help you relax.

Give yourself a good laugh: Laughing is a great way to release stress. Pandora, YouTube, or other similar websites or television stations have comedy channels. If you want to laugh really hard, tune in and listen to a few jokes or a full-length, stand-up comedy routine. Laughing activates endorphins in your brain and lowers cortisol, which is the stress hormone. The combination of the two combats stress at the chemical level and can turn your frown upside down!

Listen to soothing music or sounds: Music and sounds of nature can lower your blood pressure and heart rate. We have made it a habit of having classical music playing softly in the background in our house. The kids can concentrate better, we are more at peace, and we find it very soothing. Another option is to play sounds of nature. For example, water sounds have been found to relax the mind. Listen to the sounds of the ocean or a stream, and picture being there and watching the water move.

Get up and move: Moving your body is a key to good health and happiness. You don't have to sign up for a marathon to get the benefits of exercise. Sign up for a yoga class, go for a jog, go for a walk on the beach or a hike in the woods, ask a friend to play a sport (tennis, golf, bowling, etc.), or walk up and down the steps in your office or house. Just move your body, and get your blood moving. It's great for your heart and great for your mood.

Have sex: Sex combats stress and does so much more! It has all the benefits wrapped up in one.

This category deserves a lot of attention and is lacking in the lives of many. Sex increases the antibodies you need to fight viruses and germs. It boosts your immune system, increases blood flow to parts of the anatomy that make sex feel better and more enjoyable, strengthens the pelvic floor, improves bladder control, and decreases blood pressure. It is also a form of exercise and it burns calories, increases your heart rate, helps balance your hormone levels, improves sleep, and reduces stress. Orgasm and stimulation can actually block pain. And, sex increases self-esteem and happiness.

The best way to deal with your stress is to use all of the methods above. There will be situations where one may be easier to implement than another. However, you can make it a habit of using every method at some point during the course of a week. The more time you spend using these methods to stay relaxed, the less time stress can get into your head and body leaving you overwhelmed. Stress is a huge trigger for AF, and the key is to manage it before it gets out of control.

Conclusion

"Prayer indeed is good, but while calling on the gods a man should himself lend a hand."

- Hippocrates

Atrial fibrillation is a challenge that you can overcome. I expect you now have a better understanding of AF that will make your mission a success. You are now able to recognize the symptoms, causes, and triggers. You also now know what types of doctors you may seek and what treatment options you may be interested in exploring. I am confident that you are keenly aware of how this condition influences your risk of stroke, and I pray you are motivated to take action.

Since AF is primarily brought on by our lifestyle choices, there are three critical things I want you to immediately do at home: begin eating heart-healthy meals, add simple exercise to your daily routine, and begin utilizing stress relief techniques. Be strong and stop doing things and eating things that are making this condition worse. Believe in yourself, honor the gift of your body, and make changes that will allow you to feel proud. And, please don't be afraid to make an appointment with a doctor. The combination of at-home strategies and professional care can put your life back on track before you know it!

I want you to be free of the worry, anger, stress and fear associated with your AF. My hope and dream is that this book will help you achieve that freedom.

Lose the bad habits, be thankful for a renewed sense of knowledge and hope, and fill your life with the positive energy your heart requires to beat on, in a normal rhythm, for the rest of your life.

Best wishes on your mission—it is critical!

Appendix

AFstrokeRisk Journal

Grocery lists, To-do lists, Bucket lists...they're all useful for one reason. When one has written down, in list form, items that should be taken care of, there is a greater likelihood of those items getting checked off. When you write down a list of things you need before heading into the grocery store, you usually come home with everything you needed. A to-do list keeps you on track more than on the days you try to accomplish everything by just randomly remembering what needs to get done. A bucket list holds hope for the future and you feel a great sense of accomplishment when you are able to cross something off. The simple act of streaming your thoughts from brain to paper frees your mind, keeps you on-task, and often relieves you from additional worry and stress.

Writing things down turns thoughts into action! Keeping a journal is also an excellent way to do this. It not only offers an opportunity to reflect on what you've done, it also provides an opportunity to plan for actions you want to take going forward.

For this reason, I developed the AFstrokeRisk journal pages. This is the most powerful hands-on tool available for keeping track of the influences and triggers affecting your atrial fibrillation. This journal will turn your thoughts into action. The journal pages will be your place to document the activities of your day. Your journal will help you discover what may be contributing to your atrial fibrillation, help you set goals for tomorrow, and even draw a positive connection to the parts of your day for which you are most grateful.

You have gained a lot of insight in this book. You are now acutely aware that your lifestyle influences your AF. The goal of this journal is to help you see patterns, such as how certain foods, beverages and habits can lead to days with more AF, or simply further aggravate the AF you experience already on a regular basis.

Ultimately, this journal is meant to take you from being controlled by AF to taking control of the parts of your life that may be contributing to your AF and your risk of stroke.

This journal will also be a great resource to share with your doctor, clinician and/or nutritionist. In addition to the changes you make in your life, your medical and wellness professionals may have additional insight or explanation that will further assist you in managing your AF. By sharing the information, he/she may identify certain habits or patterns that you may not have realized are further complicating your condition.

Journaling is also a method of stress-relief and a proven way to ensure a great night sleep. On days when you experience AF, dim the lights a bit and make journaling one of the last things you do before your head hits the pillow. By writing down your thoughts and expressing your emotions before you close your eyes – you will definitely sleep more soundly. Once you have captured your swirling thoughts on paper, to sleep you will go with a mind at peace.

In the example that follows, you'll find a journal page that has already been filled in. This is followed by 7 days of blank journal pages for you to begin documenting your days with AF. As suggested, only use this journal on the days you experience AF. If you suffer every day, then use the journal each day.

In a short time, you will likely begin to see patterns. The goals for this journal: help you cut back on the foods you know or find out are triggering your AF, eat more heart-healthy options, add exercise and methods of stress-relief to your day, limit the soda, salt, sweets, cigarettes, processed foods and alcohol, etc. and ultimately begin living a lifestyle that limits the burden of AF and helps reduce the risk of stroke.

Treat yourself to a healthy lifestyle and stop slowly destroying the body and heart you rely on every day to keep you alive. I have done it and with the AFstrokeRisk journal pages, I know you can, too!

BONUS **AFstrokeRisk** JOURNAL

Track Your Triggers for 7 Days

AFstrokeRisk Journal

Example

Time and Date: __9:45PM__April 14, 2017_____
Last night, I slept_____7_____ hours

Did you sleep through, or wake up? Describe your sleep:
_____ I slept from 10 until 3, got up to use the bathroom and was awake for another hour. _____

Breakfast Time: _____ 6:30 _____

Food: ___ coffee and a bagel _____

Morning snack time: _____ no snack today _____

Food: _____

Lunch Time: ____1:15_____

Food: __2 slices of pizza and a coke _____

Afternoon snack time: ___ 4:00 ___

Food: __ Piece of cake and coffee _____

Dinner Time: ____ 7:30 _____

Food: ____ Frozen dinner of pasta and meat sauce with garlic bread

Evening snack time: ___ 9:30 ____

Food: _____ bowl of ice cream _____

How much: water did you drink today?: __ 2 glasses ____

How much soda did you drink today? __ 4 glasses _____

How much coffee, tea or other caffeinated beverages?_____
2 cups of coffee and 3 energy drinks _____

How many alcoholic drinks did you have today? _____
3 glasses of wine ____

How many cigarettes? __ 8 __

Physical exercise (what activity): _____ Went for a walk at lunch _____

Time of exercise: ____ 1:00 ____ - __ 1:15 _____

Relaxing and Rejuvenating exercise (yoga, meditation, prayer): _____ pray before bed _____

Duration of time doing yoga, meditating, praying: _____
5 minutes _____ minutes or hours

Description and times of stressful events: ____ My boss yelled at me around 2. I argued with my sister at 7 before dinner. My mother called at 9 and said she is sick. I weighed myself tonight and gained 3 pounds. ___

What time(s) did you experience atrial fibrillation today: 3-4:30 and 8-9:30 _____

How did you feel during the episode(s): ____ Racing heart, light headed, chest is pounding, upset, helpless, scared, and lonely _____

Enter your thoughts and comments about today: _____ I can't wait to go to sleep. I want a new job. _____

Today, I am grateful for: _____ My friend Pat. I love my cat. The sun was shining and I enjoyed my walk. I also saw a job on-line that I am interested in. _____

My goals for tomorrow are:

1. ___ eat better ___

2. ___ sign up for the yoga class on-line ___

3. ___ visit my mom ___

Time and Date: _____

Last night, I slept_____ hours

Did you sleep through, or wake up? Describe your sleep:

_____

_____

Breakfast Time: _____

Food: _____

_____

Morning snack time: _____

Food: _____

_____

Lunch Time: _____

Food: _____

_____

Afternoon snack time: _____

Food: _____

_____

Dinner Time: _____

Food: _____

_____

Evening snack time: _____

Food: _____

_____

How much water did you drink today?: _____

_____ glasses, ounces or liters

How much soda did you drink today? _____

_____ glasses, ounces or liters

How much coffee, tea or other caffeinated beverages?

_____

How many alcoholic drinks did you have today? _____

How many cigarettes? _____

Physical exercise (what activity): _____

_____

Time of exercise: _____ - _____

Relaxing and Rejuvenating exercise (yoga, meditation, prayer): _____

Duration of relaxing and rejuvenating exercise: _____

_____ minutes or hours

Description and times of stressful events: _____

_____

_____

_____

_____

_____

What time(s) did you experience atrial fibrillation today:

_____

How did you feel during the episode(s): _____

_____

_____

Enter your thoughts and comments about today: _____

_____

Today, I am grateful for: _____

_____

_____

My goals for tomorrow are:

1. _____

2. _____.

3. _____

Time and Date: _____

Last night, I slept_____ hours

Did you sleep through, or wake up? Describe your sleep:

_____

_____

Breakfast Time: _____

Food: _____

_____

Morning snack time: _____

Food: _____

_____

Lunch Time: _____

Food: _____

_____

Afternoon snack time: _____

Food: _____

_____

Dinner Time: _____

Food: _____

_____

Evening snack time: _____

Food: _____

_____

How much water did you drink today?: _____

_____ glasses, ounces or liters

How much soda did you drink today? _____

_____ glasses, ounces or liters

How much coffee, tea or other caffeinated beverages?

_____

How many alcoholic drinks did you have today? _____

How many cigarettes? _____

Physical exercise (what activity): _____

_____

Time of exercise: _____ - _____

Relaxing and Rejuvenating exercise (yoga, meditation, prayer): _____

Duration of relaxing and rejuvenating exercise: _____

_____ minutes or hours

Description and times of stressful events: _____

_____

_____

_____

_____

_____

What time(s) did you experience atrial fibrillation today:

_____

How did you feel during the episode(s): _____

_____

_____

Enter your thoughts and comments about today: _____

_____

Today, I am grateful for: _____

_____

_____

My goals for tomorrow are:

1. _____

2. _____

3. _____

Time and Date: _____

Last night, I slept_____ hours

Did you sleep through, or wake up? Describe your sleep:

_____

_____

Breakfast Time: _____

Food: _____

_____

Morning snack time: _____

Food: _____

_____

Lunch Time: _____

Food: _____

_____

Afternoon snack time: _____

Food: _____

_____

Dinner Time: _____

Food: _____

_____

Evening snack time: _____

Food: _____

_____

How much water did you drink today?: _____

_____ glasses, ounces or liters

How much soda did you drink today? _____

_____ glasses, ounces or liters

How much coffee, tea or other caffeinated beverages?

_____

How many alcoholic drinks did you have today? _____

How many cigarettes? _____

Physical exercise (what activity): _____

_____

Time of exercise: _____ - _____

Relaxing and Rejuvenating exercise (yoga, meditation, prayer): _____

Duration of relaxing and rejuvenating exercise: _____

_____ minutes or hours

Description and times of stressful events: _____

_____

_____

_____

_____

_____

What time(s) did you experience atrial fibrillation today:

_____

How did you feel during the episode(s): _____

_____

_____

Enter your thoughts and comments about today: _____

_____

Today, I am grateful for: _____

_____

_____

My goals for tomorrow are:

1. _____

2. _____

3. _____

Time and Date: _____

Last night, I slept_____ hours

Did you sleep through, or wake up? Describe your sleep:

_____

_____

Breakfast Time: _____

Food: _____

_____

Morning snack time: _____

Food: _____

_____

Lunch Time: _____

Food: _____

_____

Afternoon snack time: _____

Food: _____

_____

Dinner Time: _____

Food: _____

_____

Evening snack time: _____

Food: _____

_____

How much water did you drink today?: _____

_____ glasses, ounces or liters

How much soda did you drink today? _____

_____ glasses, ounces or liters

How much coffee, tea or other caffeinated beverages?

_____

How many alcoholic drinks did you have today? _____

How many cigarettes? _____

Physical exercise (what activity): _____

_____

Time of exercise: _____ - _____

Relaxing and Rejuvenating exercise (yoga, meditation, prayer): _____

Duration of relaxing and rejuvenating exercise: _____

_____ minutes or hours

Description and times of stressful events: _____

_____

_____

_____

_____

_____

What time(s) did you experience atrial fibrillation today:

_____

How did you feel during the episode(s): _____

_____

_____

Enter your thoughts and comments about today: _____

_____

Today, I am grateful for: _____

_____

_____

My goals for tomorrow are:

1. _____

2. _____

3. _____

Time and Date: _____

Last night, I slept_____ hours

Did you sleep through, or wake up? Describe your sleep:

_____

_____

Breakfast Time: _____

Food: _____

_____

Morning snack time: _____

Food: _____

_____

Lunch Time: _____

Food: _____

_____

Afternoon snack time: _____

Food: _____

_____

Dinner Time: _____

Food: _____

_____

Evening snack time: _____

Food: _____

_____

How much water did you drink today?: _____

_____ glasses, ounces or liters

How much soda did you drink today? _____

_____ glasses, ounces or liters

How much coffee, tea or other caffeinated beverages?

_____

How many alcoholic drinks did you have today? _____

How many cigarettes? _____

Physical exercise (what activity): _____

_____

Time of exercise: _____ - _____

Relaxing and Rejuvenating exercise (yoga, meditation, prayer): _____

Duration of relaxing and rejuvenating exercise: _____

_____ minutes or hours

Description and times of stressful events: _____

_____

_____

_____

_____

_____

What time(s) did you experience atrial fibrillation today:

_____

How did you feel during the episode(s): _____

_____

_____

Enter your thoughts and comments about today: _____

_____

Today, I am grateful for: _____

_____

_____

My goals for tomorrow are:

1. _____

2. _____

3. _____

Time and Date: _____

Last night, I slept_____ hours

Did you sleep through, or wake up? Describe your sleep:

_____

_____

Breakfast Time: _____

Food: _____

_____

Morning snack time: _____

Food: _____

_____

Lunch Time: _____

Food: _____

_____

Afternoon snack time: _____

Food: _____

_____

Dinner Time: _____

Food: _____

_____

Evening snack time: _____

Food: _____

_____

How much water did you drink today?: _____

_____ glasses, ounces or liters

How much soda did you drink today? _____

_____ glasses, ounces or liters

How much coffee, tea or other caffeinated beverages?

_____

How many alcoholic drinks did you have today? _____

How many cigarettes? _____

Physical exercise (what activity): _____

_____

Time of exercise: _____ - _____

Relaxing and Rejuvenating exercise (yoga, meditation, prayer): _____

Duration of relaxing and rejuvenating exercise: _____

_____ minutes or hours

Description and times of stressful events: _____

_____

_____

_____

_____

_____

What time(s) did you experience atrial fibrillation today:

_____

How did you feel during the episode(s): _____

_____

_____

Enter your thoughts and comments about today: _____

_____

Today, I am grateful for: _____

_____

_____

My goals for tomorrow are:

1. _____

2. _____

3. _____

Time and Date: _____

Last night, I slept_____ hours

Did you sleep through, or wake up? Describe your sleep:

_____

_____

Breakfast Time: _____

Food: _____

_____

Morning snack time: _____

Food: _____

_____

Lunch Time: _____

Food: _____

_____

Afternoon snack time: _____

Food: _____

_____

Dinner Time: _____

Food: _____

_____

Evening snack time: _____

Food: _____

_____

How much water did you drink today?: _____

_____ glasses, ounces or liters

How much soda did you drink today? _____

_____ glasses, ounces or liters

How much coffee, tea or other caffeinated beverages?

_____

How many alcoholic drinks did you have today? _____

How many cigarettes? _____

Physical exercise (what activity): _____

_____

Time of exercise: _____ - _____

Relaxing and Rejuvenating exercise (yoga, meditation, prayer): _____

Duration of relaxing and rejuvenating exercise: _____

_____ minutes or hours

Description and times of stressful events: _____

_____

_____

_____

_____

_____

What time(s) did you experience atrial fibrillation today:

_____

How did you feel during the episode(s): _____

_____

_____

Enter your thoughts and comments about today: _____

_____

Today, I am grateful for: _____

_____

_____

My goals for tomorrow are:

1. _____

2. _____

3. _____

27395252R00061

Printed in Great Britain
by Amazon